Nuclear Medicine Exam Questions

Andrew Kim, M.D.

ISBN 978-0-7414-1519-6

Published by:

INFINITY
PUBLISHING.COM

INFINITY PUBLISHING
1094 New DeHaven Street, Suite 100
West Conshohocken, PA 19428-2713
Toll-free (877) BUY BOOK
Local Phone (610) 941-9999
Fax (610) 941-9959
Info@buybooksontheweb.com
www.buybooksontheweb.com

Printed in the United States of America

Published July 2013

I would like to dedicate this book to my loving wife, Susy, and to my parents, YB and YY Kim. I would also like to thank my mentors, Dr. Ronald L. Van Heertum and Dr. Rashid Fawwaz of Columbia-Presbyterian Medical Center (New York, NY), and Dr. E. Stephen Amis and Dr. Leonard M. Freeman of Montefiore Medical Center (Bronx, NY).

This short book was written primarily for senior medical students rotating through nuclear medicine, residents-in-training, and fellows, in nuclear medicine and diagnostic radiology, who are studying for exams and tests. It may also be useful for those physicians who have completed their training, but would like a cursory review of testable subject matter. This book is not a substitute for any textbook, nor is it a complete review of nuclear medicine. It should be used in conjunction with other examination books, lectures and texts. The format is both multiple choice and true/false. Answers are conveniently supplied immediately following each question.

The following are 209 questions (multiple choice, and T/F). The questions are random and are not categorically grouped.

Instructions. Choose the single **BEST** answer.

1. If a radionuclide has a biological half-life of 3 hours, and a physical half-life of 6 hours, the effective half-life is:

   a. 2 hours
   b. 3 hours
   c. 4 hours
   d. 6 hours
   e. 9 hours

   Answer: (A) 2 hours. $1/T_e = 1/T_b + 1/T_p$.

2. The legal limit for molybdenum breakthrough (per mCi of 99m-Tc) is:

   a. 0.03 microcuries
   b. 0.15 microcuries
   c. 0.15 millicuries
   d. 0.3 millicuries
   e. 1.0 millicuries

   Answer: (B) 0.15 microcuries.

3. 15 millicuries of 99-Mo is equal to how many MBq?:

   a. 15 MBq
   b. 155 MBq
   c. 555 MBq
   d. 1500 MBq
   e. none of the above

   Answer: (C) 555 MBq; 1.0 mCi = 37 MBq.

4. If the true positive value is 10, the false negative value is 5, false positive value is 15, and the true negative value is 20, the accuracy is:

a. 0.2
b. 0.4
c. 0.6
d. 1.0
e. 50

Answer: (C) 0.6. Accuracy is (TP+TN) / (TP+FP+TN+FN).

5. Background radiation in the United States is approximately:

a. 160 mrem
b. 360 mrem
c. 760 mrem
d. 1500 mrem
e. 1800 mrem

Answer: (B) 360 mrem

6. Radium (226-Ra) has a half-life of:

a. 4 days
b. 8 days
c. 420 days
d. 1420 years
e. 1620 years

Answer: (E) 1620 years. Radon, not radium, has a half-life of approximately 4 days. Radon has been associated with lung cancer. It is an inhaled alpha-emitting daughter product.

7. What is the minimum dose to induce cataract formation?

a. 0.5 Sv
b. 2.0 Sv
c. 3.5 Sv
d. 4.0 Sv
e. 6.0 Sv

Answer: (B) 2.0 Sv. Note that 1 Sv = 100 rem. Note that cancer is a stochastic effect (the probability of occurrence increases as the dose increases), while cataracts are non-stochastic /deterministic (the effects are not seen below a certain threshold level).

8. The yearly permissible radiation whole body dose to radiation workers is:

a. 0.5 rem/year
b. 1.0 rem/year
c. 3.0 rem/year
d. 5.0 rem/year
e. 50 rem/year

Answer: (D) 5 rem/year. The maximum permissible dose for a pregnant radiation worker, however, is 0.5 rem for the gestation period, or < 0.05 rems per month.

9. With respect to acute radiation sickness, the gastrointestinal (GI) syndrome occurs at approximately:

a. 50 rads
b. 100 rads
c. 300 rads
d. 400 rads
e. 1000 rads

Answer: (E) The GI syndrome occurs at approximately 600-1000 rads. The Center for Disease Control (CDC) states that the syndrome will occur with a dose of 1,000 to 10,000 rads. Bone marrow suppression occurs at approximately 100 rads (the CDC states 70 –1000, and even as low as 30), while the CNS syndrome occurs at levels greater than 2000 (to 5000) rads. Note that 100 rads equals 1 Gray.

10. The minimum lethal dose in man is approximately:

a. 2 rem
b. 20 rem
c. 200 rem
d. 250 rem
e. 450 rem

Answer: (C) 200 rem.

11. A misadministration is:

a. a diagnostic dose of greater than 10% of the prescribed dose
b. a diagnostic dose of greater than 25% of the prescribed dose
c. a therapeutic dose greater than 10% of the prescribed dose
d. a therapeutic dose greater than 25% of the prescribed dose
e. a therapeutic dose of greater than 15% of the prescribed dose, or a diagnostic dose of greater than 30%

Answer: (C) A therapeutic dose greater than 10% of the prescribed dose; or a diagnostic dose of greater than 50% of the prescribed dose.

12. With respect to the Schilling test, etiologies of false low serum B_{12} levels include all, except:

a. multiple myeloma
b. third trimester pregnancy
c. anti-convulsants
d. severe liver disease
e. megaloblastic anemia secondary to folate deficiency

Answer: (D) Severe liver disease is a cause for false *normal* B_{12} level.

13. The following may cause secondary polycythemia, except:

a. pulmonary disease
b. malignancy
c. sleep apnea
d. cigarette smoking
e. all of the above are true

Answer: (E) All of the choices are causes of secondary polycythemia.

14. With respect to the dose calibrator, linearity is:

a. checked daily
b. weekly
c. quarterly
d. annually
e. at installation and then weekly

Answer: (C) Linearity is checked at installation, and then quarterly. Constancy is checked daily. Accuracy is checked at installation and then annually. Geometry is checked at installation.

15. Collimator resolution improves:

a. as the effective length of the collimator holes decreases
b. as the diameter of the collimator holes decreases
c. as the distance between the collimator and object increases
d. as the distance between the collimator and object decreases
e. a and b

Answer: (D) Collimator resolution improves as the distance between the collimator and object decreases.

16. Center of Rotation (COR) artifacts typically have which kind of an appearance?

a. ring-like
b. linear
c. triangular
d. corrugated-like
e. ovoid

Answer: (A) Ring-like, or "comet-tail."

17. The Critical Organ for Gallium is:

a. urinary bladder
b. kidney
c. stomach
d. spleen
e. distal colon

Answer: (E) Distal colon.

18. The critical organ for F-18 fluoro-deoxyglucose is:

a. urinary bladder
b. kidney
c. stomach
d. spleen
e. proximal colon

Answer: (A) Urinary bladder.

19. The Critical Organ for 99m-Tc MDP is:

a. urinary bladder
b. kidney
c. stomach
d. spleen
e. bone

Answer: (A) Urinary bladder.

20. The limulus test is used to detect the presence of pyrogens:

a. chemical purity
b. radionuclide purity
c. radiochemical purity
d. sterility
e. none of the above

Answer: (D) Sterility. The test utilizes an agent derived from the horseshoe crab.

21. The most radiosensitive phase is:

a. Metaphase
b. Anaphase
c. Telophase
d. Interphase
e. Prophase

Answer: (A) Metaphase.

22. The following are produced in a cyclotron, except:

a. 131-Iodine
b. 201-Thalium
c. 123-Iodine
d. 111-Indium
e. 67-Gallium

Answer: (A) 131-Iodine is a fission product; 133-Xenon is another fission product.

23. In beta particle emission:

a. Z increases by 1, and N decreases by 1.
b. No change in Z, and in N.
c. Z increases by 4, and N decreases by 2.
d. Z increases by 2, and N decreases by 4.
e. Z decreases by 1, and N increases by 1.

Answer: (A) Z increases by 1, and N decreases by 1.

24. If you had 10 mCi of 99m-Tc at 10:00 am on Day 1, how much would remain at 10:00 am on Day 2?

a. 0.21 mCi
b. 0.31 mCi
c. 0.41 mCi
d. 0.63 mCi
e. 1.51 mCi

Answer: (D) $A=A_0e^{(-0.693/T_{1/2})*(t)}$; $T_{1/2}$=6 hrs, t=24 hrs; A_0=10.

25. The half-life of Krypton-81m is:

a. 0.13 seconds
b. 1.3 seconds
c. 13 seconds
d. 13 minutes
e. 6 hours

Answer: (C) 13 seconds. The gamma keV is 191.

26. The principle gamma photons of 67-Gallium include all, except:

a. 93 keV
b. 159 keV
c. 184 keV
d. 296 keV
e. 388 keV

Answer: (B) 159 keV is for 123-Iodine. 67-Gallium gamma photons are approximately 90, 190, 290, and 390 keV.

27. With respect to the pulse height analyzer, a 20% symmetric window for a 140-keV photopeak:

a. 28 to 168
b. 126 to 154
c. 112 to 168
d. 120 to 160
e. 128 to 168

Answer: (B) 126 to 154, or 140-10%, and 140+10%

28. The binary number 10001 in the decimal system is:

a. 12
b. 14
c. 16
d. 17
e. 20

Answer: (D) $(1 \times 2^4) + (0 \times 2^3) + (0 \times 2^2) + (0 \times 2^1) + (1 \times 2^0) = 17$

29. With respect to gamma camera quality control, spatial resolution should be checked:

a. daily
b. weekly
c. monthly
d. quarterly
e. yearly

Answer: (B) Weekly. Uniformity and window setting are checked daily. Spatial resolution and linearity are checked weekly.

30. Which one of the following is true?

a. PET has worse spatial resolution than SPECT
b. In PET, lead collimation is not needed.
c. When a positron annihilates, two 5.11 keV photons are emitted.
d. 15-Oxygen and 12-Carbon are both cyclotron produced
e. PET radionuclides are long-lived.

Answer: (B) In PET, lead collimation is not needed. It utilizes electronic collimation instead. Without lead collimation, the system sensitivity is able to be increased.

31. Which accumulates within the choroid plexus?

a. 99m-Tc DTPA
b. 99m-Tc pertechnetate
c. 99m-Tc glucoheptonate
d. both a and b
e. all of the above

Answer: (B) 99m-Tc pertechnetate.

32. 99m-Tc RBC scintigraphy has a positive predictive value of approximately:

a. 25%
b. 50%
c. 65%
d. 80%
e. 100%

Answer: (E) 99m-Tc RBC scintigraphy has a very high positive predictive value approaching 100%. Medications which may reduce red blood cell imaging include digoxin, heparin, propranolol, doxorubicin, and methyldopa.

33. MIBG cannot be used in:

a. carcinoid
b. pheochromocytoma
c. paraganglioma
d. neuroblastoma
e. MIBG can be used in all.

Answer: (E) MIBG (metaiodobenzylguanidine) can be used in all the above mentioned tumors. Both MIBG and Octreoscan © have high sensitivity for pheochromocytoma.

34. What is the approximate percentage of MDP that localizes to bone?

a. 10%
b. 25%
c. 50%
d. 75%
e. 99%

Answer: (C) 50% of injected MDP localizes to bone.

35. Which one of the following does can metastasize to bone?

a. prostate
b. breast
c. renal
d thyroid
e. all of the above may metastasize to bone

Answer: (E) All of the above cancers may metastasize to bone.

36. (T/F) Noncemented total hip replacements may remain hot for up to 2 years on a bone scan.

Answer: True. Cemented total hip prostheses, however, should not exhibit increased uptake after 6 months. If it is, suspect loosening or infection.

37. (T/F) Dacryoscintigraphy is an application that can utilize pertechnetate.

Answer: True. The patency of the lacrimal duct can be assessed in this manner.

38. 123-Iodine commonly localizes in the following tissues, except:

a. thyroid
b. stomach
c. colon
d. liver
e. nasopharynx

Answer: (D) Liver.

39. The following are common symptoms of hypothyroidism, except for:

a. edema
b. diarrhea
c. tachycardia
d. moist skin
e. ophthalmopathy

Answer: (A) Edema is a symptom of *hyper*thyroidism.

40. With respect to the thyroid, most palpable nodules which are cold are:

a. carcinoma
b. focal thyroiditis
c. hemorrhage
d. abscess
e. adenomas

Answer: (E) Most are adenomas or colloid cysts, approximately 85%. Carcinomas represent about 10%.

41. With respect to thyroid carcinomas, which of the following is not associated with the others?

a. male
b. sudden onset
c. hard lesion
d. younger patients
e. positive family history

Answer: (B) Sudden onset is a symptom more seen in benign disease. The other choices favor malignant thyroid involvement.

42. Leukocyte WBC imaging is not normally seen in:

a. bowel
b. spleen
c. liver
d. lung
e. bone marrow

Answer: (A) Bowel. 111-Indium leukocytes and 99m-Tc HMPAO labeled leukocytes both localize to areas of infection, abscess, and osteomyelitis. has high sensitivity and specificity. WBC imaging has been used in Crohn's disease and ulcerative colitis.

43. Matched V/Q defects are seen in all of the following except:

a. atelectasis
b. bullous disease
c. pneumonectomy
d. pneumonia
e. hypoplastic pulmonary artery

Answer: (E) Hypoplastic pulmonary artery is seen in V/Q mismatches.

44. False positive thallium studies can be seen in all except:

a. aortic valve stenosis
b. submaximal stress
c. mitral valve prolapse
d. left bundle branch block
e. Chagas disease

Answer: (B) Submaximal stress is a reason for false *negative* exams. An optimal test is when the heart rate reaches (220-patient age) x 0.85.

45. False positive HIDA studies include all, except:

a. pancreatitis
b. right lower lobe pneumonia
c. recent meal
d. pancreatitis
e. duodenal diverticulum

Answer: (E) Duodenal diverticulum is a cause for false *negative* studies.

46. In testicular imaging, a ring sign or a ring-type sign can be seen in:

a. tumor
b. abscess
c. trauma
d. late torsion
e. all of the above

Answer: (E) All of the above.

47. Focal photopenic lesions in bone scan can often be seen in the following neoplasms, except:

a. lymphoma
b. renal
c. thyroid
d. neuroblastoma
e. prostate

Answer: (E) Prostate cancer most often exhibits *increased* activity.

48. (T/F) Mild Parkinson's disease has a similar appearance as Alzheimer's disease on brain scans.

Answer: False. *Severe/advanced* Parkinson's has a similar appearance as Alzheimer's disease on brain scans.

49. Picks's Disease is characterized by hypoperfusion in:

a. occipital
b. frontal
c. cerebellum
d. parietal

Answer: (B) Frontal lobe. Pick's disease is a rare dementia that commonly presents in patients before age 60. It is associated with frontal and temporal lobe atrophy. Symptoms include lack of spontaneity, difficulty in thinking or concentrating, loss of memory, and speech disturbances.

50. Which of the following has approximately 100% tubular uptake?

a. Tc-99m DTPA
b. Tc-99m MAG3
c. I-131 OIH
d. I-123 OIH
e. Tc-99m DMSA

Answer: (B) Tc-99m MAG3.

51. .(T/F) I-125 orthoiodohippurate (OIH) can be used to quantify effective renal plasma flow.

Answer: True.

52. (T/F) Acute rejection in renal transplantation is typically seen in 1-5 days.

Answer: False. *Accelerated* rejection is seen in 1-5 days. Acute rejection is seen after 5 days, commonly during the first 3 months.

53. (T/F) Torsion of the testicular appendage is commonly seen in men ages 21-35.

Answer: False. Torsion of the testicular appendage is commonly seen in boys 7-14 years old. Radionuclide exam may be normal or may demonstrate subtle activity.

54. Induction of thyrotoxicosis in a euthyroid patient after large amounts of iodine exposure is seen in:

a. Jod-Basedow phenomenon
b. De Quervain's disease
c. Plummer's disease
d. Wolff-Chaikoff
e. Marine-Lenhart syndrome

Answer: (A) Jod-Basedow phenomenon. The Wolff-Chaikoff effect is when large doses of iodide are administered acutely, inducing a relative or absolute inhibition of iodination of thyroglobulin. Beyond a critical dose level, larger doses of iodide may lead to progressively smaller quantities of iodinated thyroglobulin within the gland. Plummer's disease is a nodular toxic goiter. The coexistence of a TSH dependent functioning nodule(s) and Grave's disease is referred to as Marine-Lenhart syndrome.

55. The following drugs can interfere with MIBG uptake, except:

a. reserpine
b. cocaine
c. labetolol
d. tricyclic antidepressants
e. digoxin

Answer: (E) Digoxin.

56. (T/F) The effective half-life can be longer than the biological half-life.

Answer: (F) The effective half-life is always shorter than the biological half-life or the physical half-life. $1/T_e = 1/T_b + 1/T_p$.

57. What is the maximum number of electrons that can occupy the outermost shell of an atom?

a. 2
b. 4
c. 6
d. 8
e. 10

Answer: (D) 8

58. (T/F) Normal-pressure hydrocephalus (NPH) manifests clinically with dementia, vertigo, and constipation.

Answer: (F) NPH manifests as dementia, ataxia, and incontinence. The gold standard for establishing the diagnosis is a clinical response to cerebrospinal fluid tap.

59. The sensitivity of gallium-67 is highest in detecting which tumor?

a. Non-Hodgkin's disease
b. Hodgkin's disease
c. Melanoma
d. Lung cancer
e. Hepatocellular carcinoma

Answer: (B) The sensitivity is reported to be greater than 90% for Hodgkin's disease.

60. With regards to Hodgkin's disease, the prognosis is highest for which subgroup?

a. lymphocyte depleted
b. mixed cellularity
c. nodular sclerosis
d. lymphocyte predominant

Answer: (D) Lymphocyte predominant. The prognosis is poor for lymphocyte depleted. Hodgin's lymphoma has a bimodal age distribution with peaks in the mid-late 20s, and late adulthood. Hodgkin's disease is a lymphoma characterized by a pleomorphic cellular infiltrate with multinucleated giant cells (Reed-Sternberg cells).

61. (T/F) Hodgkin's disease spreads in a contiguous nodal spread.

Answer: True. Hodgkin's disease spreads contiguously, while as Non-Hodgkin's disease is discontiguous.

62. (T/F) Kaposi's sarcoma is Ga-67 positive but Tl-201 negative.

Answer: False. Kaposi's sarcoma is Ga-67 *negative*, but Tl-201 *positive*. The most common site for KS is on the skin but it also affects internal organs, such as the lymph nodes, the lungs and parts of the digestive system.

63. (T/F) Radiation therapy and chemotherapy usually increases tumor uptake of fluorodeoxyglucose.

Answer: False. Radiation therapy and chemotherapy may decrease tumor uptake of fluorodeoxyglucose.

64. (T/F) Colon cancer is the leading cause of death in the United States for both men and women.

Answer: False. Lung cancer is the leading cause. Lung cancer is the most common form of cancer diagnosed in the United States and a major cause of death. Lung cancer accounts for 14% of all cancers and 28% of all cancer deaths.

65. (T/F) CEA-Scan © has higher HAMA than OncoScint ©.

Answer: False. The HAMA for CEA-Scan © is <1%, while for OncoScint ©, it is about 40%. The human patient mounts an immune response against the murine antibodies. Oncoscint specifically targets the cell surface mucin-like glycoprotein antigen TAG-72, seen in ovarian and colorectal carcinomas.

66. (T/F) In-111 Prostascint © reacts with prostate specific antigen (PSA).

Answer: False. In -111 Prostascint © reacts with prostate specific *membrane* antigen (PSMA).

67. In-111 Octreoscan © has the highest sensitivity for which of the following?

a. carcinoid
b. gastrinoma
c. medullary thyroid carcinoma
d. glucagonoma
e. insulinoma

Answer: (B) Out of the above choices, In-111 Octreoscan has the highest sensitivity for gastrinoma, approximately 95%. Gastrinomas are rare endocrine tumors and commonly present with severe recurrent peptic ulcer disease. More than 60% of gastrinomas are cancerous and the tumor eventually metastasizes to the liver and other viscera. The initial clinical manifestations appear most commonly in patients from 30–50 years of age. Gastrinomas cause the Zollinger Ellison syndrome. Almost 25% of gastrinoma patients have multiple tumors as part of the MEN syndromes.

68. For an adult with a bilirubin of 10 mg/dl, an accepted usual dose for Tc-99m mebrofenin is:

a. 1.0 mCi
b. 2.5 mCi
c. 5.0 mCi
d. 10.0 mCi
e. 25 mCi

Answer: (D) 10.0 mCi (370 MBq).

69. Which of the following is not an action of cholecystokinin?

a. stimulates intestinal motility
b. stimulates hepatic bile secretion
c. stimulates pancreatic enzyme secretion
d. stimulates gastric emptying
e. promotes gallbladder contraction

Answer: (D) Cholecystokinin inhibits gastric emptying.

70. (T/F) The "rim sign" in hepotobiliary imaging is seen in approximately 60% of patients with acute cholecystitis.

Answer: False. It is seen in only about 25%. The "rim sign" is increased activity in the region of the gallbladder fossa, and is associated with patients in the later stages of acute cholecystitis (ie. necrosis, gangrene).

71. (T/F) With respect to biliary atresia, pretreatment with phenobarbital before Tc-99m HIDA imaging is maximized by activating the liver excretory enzymes.

Answer: True. The dose is 5 mg/kg/day for 5 days before imaging.

72. (T/F) The characteristic finding with focal nodular hyperplasia (FNH) in cholescintigraphy is decreased blood flow, prompt hepatic uptake, and prompt clearance.

Answer: False. The characteristic finding with focal nodular hyperplasia (FNH) in cholescintigraphy is *increased* blood flow, prompt hepatic uptake, and delayed clearance. FNH is usually an asymptomatic, incidentally discovered lesion. It is considered a benign tumor, and is usually solitary, although it can present as multiple lesions in up to 10-20% of patients.

73. (T/F) Strontium-89 is accumulated in metabolically active bone because of its chemical similarity to phosphate.

Answer: False. Strontium-89 is accumulated in metabolically active bone because of its chemical similarity to *calcium*. Strontium-89 is used to treat painful bone metastases. It provides local radiation at the site of these lesions. Strontium (beta decay) has a physical half-life of 50.5 days.

74. (T/F) All I-131 imaging and therapy of thyroid carcinoma should be carried out in the setting of low TSH levels.

Answer: False. All I-131 imaging and therapy of thyroid carcinoma should be carried out in the setting of *high* TSH levels. T4 should be discontinued approximately 6 weeks before, and replaced with T3. T3 is discontinued approximately 2 weeks before imaging or therapy.

75. Using I-131-19-iodocholesterol (NP-59), adrenal cortical carcinoma may show which of the following:

a. bilateral symmetric increased activity
b. bilateral nonvisualization
c. mildly asymmetrical activity
d. unilateral activity

Answer: (B) Bilateral nonvisualization. NP-59, a cholesterol analog, is useful in the evaluation of incidentally detected adrenal masses (incidentalomas) and hyperaldosteronism.

76. P-32 is used in all of the following except:

a. polycythemia vera
b. hemophilic arthropathy
c. craniopharyngioma
d. disseminated ovarian cancer
e. non-metastasized melanoma

Answer: (E) Non-metastasized melanoma. P-32 (beta decay) has been used to treat diseases such as polycythemia vera, lymphocytic leukemia, myelogenous leukemia, non-Hodgkin's lymphoma, Hodgins disease, thrombocytopenia, and as a palliative treatment of metastatic bone cancer, among others. It has a half-life of 14.3 days.

77. (T/F) Herpes brain infection classically demonstrates increased activity, when utilizing Tc-99m DTPA, in the high parietal lobes.

Answer: False. Herpes brain infection classically demonstrates increased activity, when utilizing Tc-99m DTPA, in the *temporal* lobes.

78. (T/F) When performing a V/Q scan, Xe-133 ventilation is performed after Tc-99m MAA perfusion.

Answer: False. The 80 keV predominant energy peak of Xe-133 necessitates that ventilation imaging be performed *before* perfusion.

79. In cardiac imaging, ideally, the double product should be at least:

a. 1800
b. 2400
c. 7600
d. 15500
e. 24000

Answer: (E) The double product is the product of peak heart rate and peak systolic pressure. Ideally, it should be 24000 or more.

80. (T/F) Tc-99m teboroxime has slow clearance from the myocardium.

Answer: False. Its rapid clearance distinguishes this neutral lipid soluble agent from thallium or sestamibi.

81. (T/F) In cardiac scintigraphy, heating is necessary for preparation of Tc-99m tetrofosmin.

Answer: False. Heating is not necessary for preparation of Tc-99m tetrofosmin.

82. (T/F) With respect to cardiac gated blood pool imaging, the in vivo method produces labeling efficiencies in the 95% range.

Answer: False. The in vivo method produces labeling efficiencies in the 80-90% range, while the *modified in vivo* method produces labeling efficiencies in the 95% range. The in vitro method produces labeling efficiencies greater than 95%.

83. (T/F) Gated blood pool imaging is often utilized in patients receiving doxorubicin.

Answer: True. Doxorubicin (Adriamycin©). Moderate cardiotoxicity is a drop in the LVEF of more than 15 points, or an absolute left ventricular ejection fraction of less than 45%.

84. (T/F) Sensitivity is highest in assessing necrotic myocardium with In-111-labeled antimyosin at 6-12 hours following infarction.

Answer: False. Sensitivity is highest in assessing necrotic myocardium with In-111-labeled antimyosin at *24-48* hours following infarction.

85. (T/F) Indium-111 is preferred over Gallium-67 for vertebral osteomyelitis.

Answer: False. Gallium-67 is preferred over Indium-111 for vertebral osteomyelitis. Ga-67 (beta decay) mimics ferric iron in uptake and distribution but does not incorporate hemoglobin.

86. (T/F) Well-differentiated papillary thyroid carcinomas tend to metastasize via lymph nodes, while follicular thyroid carcinomas tend to metastasize hematogenously.

Answer: True. Papillary tumors are the most common of all thyroid cancers , >70%. Spread to cervical lymph nodes is present in more than 50% of cases. Peak onset, ages 30 – 50.

87. (T/F) Medullary and anaplastic thyroid carcinomas commonly concentrate I-131.

Answer: False. Medullary and anaplastic thyroid carcinomas do not commonly concentrate I-131. Consequently, iodine imaging is not performed for those with medullary or anaplastic carcinomas.

88. (T/F) The "stripe sign" in lung scintigraphy refers to fluid in the interlobar fissure, causing perfusion defects.

Answer: False. The "stripe sign" refers to the border between a perfusion defect and the pleural surface of the lung. A peripheral margin of relatively preserved perfusion does not favor embolism.

89. Classically, diffuse gallium-67 uptake in the lungs can be seen the following, except :

a. pneumocystis carinii (PCP) infection
b. interstitial pneumonitis
c. cytomegolovirus (CMV) infection
d. mycobacterium avium intracellulare (MAI)

Answer: (D) Mycobacterium avium intracellulare (MAI) infection is often seen in a lobar or an asymmetric pattern with hilar lymph node involvement.

90. (T/F) 99m-Tc MAG3 will reveal better diagnostic quality than 99m-Tc DTPA during impaired renal function.

Answer: True.

91. Which of the following is not gallium-avid?

a. multiple myeloma
b. Kaposi's sarcoma
c. neuroblastoma
d. melanoma
e. rhabdomyosarcoma

Answer: (B) Kaposi's sarcoma. Multiple myeloma may be gallium-avid.

92. By modified PIOPED criteria, a small matched V/Q defects makes the likelihood of a pulmonary embolus:

a. normal
b. low
c. intermediate
d. high

Answer: (B) Low probability.

93. By modified PIOPED criteria, one moderate mismatched segmental defect with a normal chest x-ray has a probability of:

a. normal
b. low
c. intermediate
d. high

Answer: (C) Intermediate.

94. By modified PIOPED criteria, one large and one moderate mismatched segmental defect with a normal chest x-ray has a probability of:

a. normal
b. low
c. intermediate
d. high

Answer: (C) Intermediate.

95. (T/F) Patients with lymphoma typically have symmetrical hilar uptake.

Answer: False. Patients with lymphoma typically have asymmetrical hilar uptake. Sarcoid may be symmetrical.

96. (T/F) Multiple sites of focal increased gallium-67 activity in the lungs can be seen with Nocardia infection.

Answer: True. Nocardia, Actinomyces, and Aspergillus can be gallium-avid.

97. (T/F) In F-18 FDG PET imaging, a seizure focus is seen as an area of increased activity during the ictus, while in SPECT imaging, it is seen as an area of decreased activity.

Answer: False. A seizure focus is seen as an area of increased activity during the ictus in both PET and SPECT imaging.

98. Classically, decreased activity in the caudate nucleus is seen in which of the following:

a. Huntington's disease
b. Pick's disease
c. Alzheimer's disease
d. Parkinson's disease
e. Schizophrenia

Answer: (A) Huntington's disease.

99. (T/F) ACE inhibitors work by blocking the conversion of angiotensin I to angiotensin II.

Answer: True.

100. (T/F) Gender is a factor that can affect gastric emptying results.

Answer: True.

101. (T/F) For the treatment of chronic gastroparesis, domperidone works by releasing acetylcholine from the myenteric plexus.

Answer: False. Cisapride works by releasing acetylcholine from the myenteric plexus. Domperidone is a dopamine antagonist.

102. (T/F) The thicker the crystal, the better the resolution, and the better the efficiency in detecting gamma rays.

Answer: False. The thicker the crystal, the *poorer* the resolution, and the better the efficiency in detecting gamma rays.

103. (T/F) With respect to the gamma camera, the lead x-ray peak is due to primary gamma rays undergoing Compton scattering in the collimator, or the lead shielding.

Answer: False. The lead x-ray peak is due to primary gamma rays undergoing the *photoelectric effect* in the collimator, or the lead shielding.

104. (T/F) For SPECT images, filtering cannot be performed after transaxial reconstruction.

Answer: False. For SPECT images, filtering *can* be performed , during, or before, transaxial reconstruction.

105. Which of the following is NOT a typical filter used in SPECT image production?

a. Hamming
b. Parzen
c. Butterworth
d. Jaszczak
e. Hann

Answer: (D) Jaszczak is a type of phantom used in system performance. The others are commonly used filters.

106. The maximum acceptable uncorrected error in the center of rotation (COR) is how many pixels?

a. 0.1
b. 0.2
c. 0.5
d. 1.5
e. 2.5

Answer: (C) 0.5

107. (T/F) SPECT myocardial perfusion acquisition is most commonly performed over 180 degrees.

Answer: True. SPECT myocardial perfusion acquisition is most commonly performed over 180 degrees, while other types of studies are often performed over 360 degrees.

108. Functional SPECT brain perfusion imaging is often employed in the following, except:

a. transient ischemic attacks
b. Alzheimer's disease
c. brain death
d. acute trauma
e. acute stroke

Answer: (D) Acute trauma is not a common setting for the utilization of SPECT brain perfusion imaging. A CT scan would likely be warranted.

109. (T/F) With regards to PET imaging, steroids may interfere by increasing glucose metabolism in the brain.

Answer: False. Steroids may interfere by decreasing glucose metabolism in the brain.

110. (T/F) Communicating hydrocephalus classically presents scintigraphically with entry into the lateral ventricles at 4-6 hours, with persistence of lateral ventricular activity at 24-72 hours.

Answer: True. Those patients that exhibit this finding may often benefit from shunting.

111. (T/F) In regions of vascular disease, regional perfusion is enhanced after the administration of Diamox ©.

Answer: False. In regions of vascular disease, regional perfusion is worsened after the administration of Diamox.

112. In cardiac imaging, breast attenuation artifact affects which wall the most?

a. Anterior
b. Base
c. Inferior
d. Septal
e. (b) or (d) equally

Answer: (A) Anterior or lateral wall defects may occur. An elevated left hemidiaphragm may affect the inferior wall.

113. (T/F) In cardiac imaging, transient left ventricular cavity dilatation is always normal.

Answer: False. Transient left ventricular cavity dilatation can be seen in the setting of left ventricular dysfunction, or subendocardial ischemia. Fixed dilatation is seen in pre-existing cavity enlargement.

114. In a 62 year old female utilizing the Bruce protocol, the endpoint is when the heart rate reaches what number?

a. 127
b. 134
c. 149
d. 153
e. 161

Answer: (B) 134. The endpoint is reached when the patient reaches 85% of the maximum predicted heart rate. This is calculate by subtracting the patient's age from 220, and then multiplying this number by 0.85. In this example, 220-62 = 158; 158 x 0.85 = 134.

115. Left bundle-branch block can cause which finding in cardiac SPECT imaging?

a. a reversible inferior wall defect
b. a fixed anterior/apical wall defect
c. a reversible septal wall defect
d. a fixed lateral wall defect
e. a fixed septal wall defect

Answer: (C) A reversible septal wall defect.

116. Ventricular aneurysms appear as focal areas of:

a. akinesis
b. hypokinesis
c. tardokinesis
d. dyskinesis

Answer (D) Dyskinesis. The other choices can be seen in areas of scarred or injured myocardium. Akinetic means absent motion.

117. (T/F) 99m-Tc sestamibi is actively taken up by the Na^+-K^+ pump in the cells.

Answer: False. Thallium is actively taken up by the Na^+-K^+ pump in the cells. 99m-Tc sestamibi passively diffuses across the membrane.

118. (T/F) The normal right ventricular ejection fraction is approximately 35-50%.

Answer: True. The normal right ventricular ejection fraction is approximately 35-50%. A normal left ventricular ejection fraction is in the range of 55-65%.

119. In lung scintigraphy, what is the percentage of capillaries that are blocked by 99m-Tc macroaggregated albumin (MAA)?

a. 0.1%
b. 1.0%
c. 5.0%
d. 10%
e. 15%

Answer: (A) 0.1% or 1/1000.

120. A "triple match" or a ventilation-perfusion abnormality accompanied by a matching opacity is which probability of pulmonary embolism?

a. normal
b. very low
c. low
d. intermediate
e. high

Answer: (D) Intermediate probability

121. (T/F) In a patient with normal ventilation, and a total absence of the right lung on perfusion imaging, the most likely etiology is pulmonary embolus.

Answer: False. One would have to consider a large right hilar mass/neoplasm constricting the right pulmonary artery.

122. (T/F) Kidney activity on a 99mTc-MAA scan indicates a possible left-to-right shunt.

Answer: False. Kidney activity on a 99m-Tc MAA scan indicates a possible *right-to-left* shunt. One can confirm this by determining brain activity.

123. Decreased activity on a 99m-Tc sulfur colloid study can be seen in all, except:

a. hemangioma
b. cyst
c. metastatic focus
d. adenoma
e. regenerating nodule from cirrhosis

Answer: (E) Regenerating nodule from cirrhosis is associated with increased activity.

124. On a HIDA study, hepatocellular carcinoma typically will demonstrate ______ activity on the perfusion phase.

a. normal
b. increased
c. decreased

Answer: (C) Decreased on the *perfusion* phase; normal/decreased on the parenchymal phase; and delayed washout.

125. Tc-99m apcitide (AcuTect ©) is used for:

a. abscess evaluation
b. brain death
c. shunt patency
d. deep venous thrombosis
e. osteomyelitis

Answer: (D) Deep venous thrombosis. AcuTect's peptide element adheres to the GP IIb/IIIa receptor on the surface of activated platelets, which is a major component of active thrombus formation.

126. Approximately, how many people are diagnosed with lung cancer per year?

a. 50,000
b. 75,000
c. 100,000
d. 170,000
e. 420,000

Answer: (D) 170,000.

127. (T/F) The normal thyroid gland weighs 15-20 grams.

Answer: True.

128. Which of the following has been known to cause false-positive 131-Iodine scans?

a. meningioma
b. Zenker's diverticulum
c. thymus
d. gastric carcinoma
e. all of the above

Answer: (E) All of the above. Other etiologies include achalasia, and lung cancer.

129. (T/F) 111-Indium octreotide and MIBG imaging have roughly equal sensitivities in detecting pheochromocytoma.

Answer: True.

130. Which of the following are not associated with schizencephaly?

a. macrogyria
b. mental retardation
c. hemiplegia
d. seizures
e. hemiparesis

Answer: (A) Macrogyria. Schizencephaly, an extremely rare developmental disorder, is characterized by abnormal clefts, or slits, in the brain's cerebral hemispheres. The cleft is lined by gray matter. Schizencephaly is associated with *microgyria.*

131. What is the typical adult dose of 99mTc-sulfur colloid for gastroesophageal reflux scintigraphy?

a. 100 microcuries
b. 300 microcuries
c. 750 microcuries
d. 1.0 Curie
e. 1.5 Curies

Answer: (B) 300 microcuries of 99m-Tc sulfur colloid mixed with orange juice.

132. (T/F) Shin splints often appear as cortical, focal oval or fusiform activity, in a transverse distribution.

Answer: False. Stress fractures appear as cortical, focal oval or fusiform activity, in a transverse distribution.

133. Which is NOT a characteristic of Paget's disease?

a. common in the ages between 20-40
b. elevated serum alkaline phosphatase
c. has three phases: lytic, sclerotic, and mixed
d. 20% are monostotic
e. bone enlargement

Answer: (A) Paget's disease is common after the age of 40. A small percentage (<1%) may undergo malignant degeneration to osteosarcoma.

134. (T/F) With regards to the Evans neuroblastoma staging, stage IV disease is disseminated disease with skeletal metastases.

Answer: True. Stage I is confined to the structure of origin. Stage II involves tumor extension, but not across the midline. Stage III disease extends across the midline. Stage IV disease is disseminated disease with skeletal metastases.

135. (T/F) Bone scans have low yield in Stage I and II breast cancer.

Answer: True. However, some patients with poor prognostic stage II disease may benefit.

136. Which is NOT a characteristic of fibrous dysplasia?

a. congenital, nonhereditary
b. 75% are polyostotic
c. frequent sites are tibia, femur and facial bones
d. occurs during periods of bone growth
e. marrow is replaced by fibrous tissue

Answer: (B) 75% are *monostotic*. Fibrous dysplasia is a benign entity, whereby the medullary cavity is replaced by fibrous material and woven bone. They usually exhibit increased uptake on bone scans.

137. Stress myocardial perfusion imaging has a sensitivity of what percent for the detection of coronary artery disease?

a. 35%
b. 55%
c. 70%
d. 85%
e. 96%

Answer: (D) In comparison, stress echocardiography has a sensitivity of 70% for the detection of coronary artery disease.

138. (T/F) When using 99m-Tc myocardial perfusion agents, mild uptake in the lungs is indicative of left ventricular failure.

Answer: False. When using 99m-Tc myocardial perfusion agents, mild uptake in the lungs can be seen normally, as opposed to 201-thallium. 201-Thallium activity in the lungs is a sign of left ventricular decompensation, and may be a sign of multivessel coronary artery disease. A lung/myocardial activity ratio of greater than 0.5 is abnormal.

139. Which of the following statements concerning sarcoidosis is false?

a. the lung is the most involved organ
b. 75% are asymptomatic
c. 10-20 times more common in blacks than in whites
d. treatment may involve steroids
e. the Kveim test may be used for diagnosis

Answer: (B) 30% are asymptomatic.

140. In inferior vena cava obstruction, injection of 99m-Tc sulfur colloid or MAA into a lower extremity vein results in hyperactivity in which area?

a. Riedel's lobe
b. caudate lobe
c. quadrate lobe
d. pancreas
e. spleen

Answer: (C) This is because venous blood is rerouted through collateral vessels to the left umbilical vein and into the left portal vein. Budd-Chiari syndrome may demonstrate a hot *caudate* lobe.

141. (T/F) Red blood cell scintigraphy may detect a bleeding rate as low as 0.4 mL/min, while angiography requires a rate of greater than 1mL/min.

Answer: True. Red blood cell imaging is about 90% sensitive in the detection of GI bleeding.

142. A 46 year old male with Grave's disease presents to the hospital. He has an enlarged thyroid gland (approximately 60 grams). Assuming the 24 hour uptake was 52%, and 100 microcuries/gram is desired, what will be the dose of 131-I, in mCi?

a. 1.5
b. 8.8
c. 10.0
d. 11.5
e. 21.5

Answer: (D) The equation is (gram size x 100 microcuries/gram) / 24 hr. uptake. In this case, (60 grams x 100 microcuries/gram) / 0.52 = 11,539 microcuries. In mCi, this equals 11,539/1000 = 11.5 mCi. Some may opt anywhere between 50 – 200 microcuries per gram, depending on the patient and the situation.

143. Which of the following is FALSE concerning Warthin's tumor?

a. it is malignant
b. it can concentrate 99m-Tc pertechnetate
c. it accounts for 2% of all head and neck tumors
d. peak incidence is in the sixth and seventh decades of life
e. also known as papillary cystadenoma

Answer: (A) Warthin's tumor is a *benign* tumor. 5-20% are bilateral, and it occurs much more often in males than in females.

144. (T/F) With regards to vesiocoureteral reflux disease, grade II is reflux extending into the ureter and pelvicalyceal system without dilatation.

Answer: True. Grade I is reflux limited to the ureter. Grade II is reflux extending into the ureter and pelvicalyceal system without dilatation. Grade III is mild to moderate dilatation of the ureter and pelvis without forniceal blunting, while grade IV is moderate dilatation of the ureter and pelvis with obliteration of the sharp angles of the fornices. Grade V is severe dilatation of the ureter and pelvicalyceal system with loss of papillary impressions.

145. Which of the following is FALSE concerning renovascular hypertension?

a. captopril MAG-3 renogram will reveal significant cortical retention of the affected side
b. it is a common condition that occurs in 15-20% of hypertensive patients
c. captopril renography has a sensitivity of approximately 90% for the detection of renovascular hypertension
d. angiotensin I is converted to angiotensin II by ACE
e. 131-I hippuran may demonstrate a similar appearance as MAG-3

Answer: (B) Renovascular hypertension (RVH) is an uncommon condition, occurring is less than 1% of hypertensive patients.

146. (T/F) A Lasix © washout half-time of less than 10 minutes indicates no obstruction, between 10-20 minutes is indeterminate, and greater than 20 minutes suggests an obstructed system.

Answer: True. A lasix washout half-time of less than 10 minutes indicates no obstruction, between 10-20 minutes is indeterminate, and greater than 20 minutes suggests an obstructed system.

147. What is the dosage for morphine in hepatobiliary scintigraphy imaging in an adult?

a. 0.01 mg/kg
b. 0.02 mg/kg
c. 0.04 mg/kg
d. 1.00 mg/kg
e. a standard dosage of 10 mg is sufficient.

Answer: (C) The adult dosage is 0.04 mg/kg.

148. Which is true regarding 99m-Tc sulfur colloid imaging for gastrointestinal bleeding?

a. it is administered orally
b. it is cleared from the vascular system within 15-20 minutes
c. the target to background ratio is low
d. bleeding can be detected 24 hours later
e. has a higher detection rate than angiography

Answer: (B) It is cleared from the vascular system within 15-20 minutes.

148. Which is true regarding the gastric emptying test?

a. if the liquid gastric emptying test is normal, than the solid test will be normal.
b. the geometric mean is the most accurate
c. the antrum is primarily involved in liquid emptying
d. the study can be obtained optimally in the LPO position
e. not a very good test for gastroparesis

Answer: (B) The geometric mean requires both anterior and posterior acquisitions with mathematical corrections. Alternatively, the test can be performed in the LAO position. The fundus is primarily involved in liquid emptying. If the solid gastric emptying test is normal, than the liquid test will be normal. The gastric emptying test is utilized in diabetics with possible gastric outlet obstruction, or gastroparesis.

149. Which of the following is true?

a. an isoelectric flat EEG is only seen in brain death.
b. 99m-Tc DTPA is the only radiotracer used for brain death studies
c. the diagnosis is primarily a clinical one
d. cerebral blood flow can be seen in brain death
e. the "hot ear" sign has high sensitivity for brain death

Answer: (C) The diagnosis is primarily a clinical one. Barbituate use and hypothermia may also result in an isoelectric flat EEG. 99m-Tc HMPAO and ECD can also be used in brain death scintigraphy. The "hot *nose*" sign can be seen with brain death.

150. (T/F) Cyclosporin toxicity is usually seen days after renal transplantation.

Answer: False. Cyclosporin toxicity is usually occurs *months* after renal transplantation. Acute rejection, obstruction, and acute tubular necrosis (ATN) usually occurs during the first weeks after transplantation.

151. (T/F) The flare phenomenon is the time when more metastastic lesions are detected, and therefore more aggressive treatment should be employed.

Answer: False. The flare phenomenon is when there is increasing uptake on a bone scan during the treatment of metastatic disease secondary to healing of the tumor, rather than progression. It is frequently seen in prostate and breast cancers.

152. Lung uptake in a bone scan can be seen in:

a. radiation fibrosis
b. fibrothorax
c. metastatic calcification
d. metastatic osteosarcoma
e. all of the above

Answer: (E) All of the above.

153. (T/F) PET scanning is not useful in testicular carcinomas.

Answer: False. PET has a role in ascertaining the extent of viable tumor before salvage surgery in follow-up patients. It can evaluate viable tumor from scar. 1% of all cancers in men are testicular carcinomas.

154. (T/F) If gut activity is seen on a PET scan, the study is positive.

Answer: False. Gut activity is highly variable, and is often commonly seen in the stomach, duodenum, and in the colon.

155. (T/F) Metastasis may skip the expected iliac or perilumbar route in prostate cancer.

Answer: True. In fact, the first lymph node can be seen even in the supraclavicular region. However, the first lymph nodes to be involved are more often the periprostatic and obturator lymph nodes.

156. (T/F) An elevated CEA level without identified site in colon cancer is currently a reimbursable indication in PET imaging.

Answer: True. An elevated CEA level without identified site in colon cancer is currently a reimbursable indication in PET imaging. Other reimbursable indication include lymphoma, melanoma, lung nodule work-up, and esophageal cancer staging.

157. (T/F) With regards to cardiac agents, 99m-Tc tetrofosmin (© Myoview) is most similar to thallium.

Answer: False. 99m-Tc tetrofosmin is most similar to sestamibi. However, it is cleared from the lungs and liver more rapidly than sestamibi.

158. (T/F) Adenosine has a lower incidence of minor side effects than persantine.

Answer: False. Side effects with adenosine include shortness of breath, flushing, and chest pain. Also, if it infused too rapidly, transient heart block may occur.

159. With regards to bleeding scintigraphy, which is *false*:

a. a major disadvantage with the 99m-Tc sulfur colloid method is that bleeding must be active
b. a vascular blush can be seen with angiodysplasia on the flow phase
c. radiotracer activity must be seen as moving to be diagnosed as active bleeding
d. the hepatic flexure is supplied by the inferior mesenteric artery
e. the in vitro RBC kit utilizes sodium hypochlorite as an oxidizing agent

Answer: (D) The hepatic flexure is supplied by the *superior* mesenteric artery.

160. (T/F) The typical adult dose for 99m-Tc RBC gastrointestinal bleeding scintigraphy is 5 mCi.

Answer: False. The typical dose is 25 mCi for 99m-Tc RBC, and 10 mCi for 99m-Tc sulfur colloid scintigraphy.

161. (T/F) It is preferred to administer sodium perchlorate for thyroid radiation protection before a gastric scintigraphic study utilizing 99m-Tc pertechnetate.

Answer: False. Sodium perchlorate will prevent uptake in the gastric mucosa.

162. (T/F) Mean cerebral blood flow (CBF) in children is less than in a normal adult.

Answer: False. Children have a CBF of 100 ml/min/100 g, while adult mean CBF is around 50 ml/min/100 g.

163. (T/F) Cerebral blood flow can be measured by quantifying the clearance of xenon-133 from the brain.

Answer: True. Cerebral blood flow can be measured by quantifying the clearance of xenon-133 from the brain. Xenon-133, a lipid-soluble gas, diffuses rapidly into tissues. Its washout is also rapid and is directly proportional to cerebral blood flow.

164. (T/F) Gamma camera resolution is improved by using a pinhole collimator.

Answer: True. Pinhole collimation has high resolution, but poorer sensitivity, since there are fewer photons getting through.

165. A 45 year old obese female with right upper quadrant pain has a HIDA scan. After 45 minutes of sequential imaging, activity is seen in the liver, biliary tree, and in the small bowel. The next appropriate step is:

a. a fatty meal
b. reinject Tc-99m HIDA and scan for an additional 2 hours
c. morphine
d. conclude the exam
e. administer CCK

Answer: (C) Administer morphine (0.04 mg/kg, up to 4 mg), which will contract the sphincter of Oddi, and cause reflux into a patent cystic duct and gallbladder.

166. (T/F) Hypertrophic pulmonary osteoarthropathy (HPO) commonly causes linear increased activity along the shafts of primarily the mid-ulna.

Answer: False. HPO is most commonly seen in those patients with lung cancer. On bone scans, it may appear as linear increased activity along the shafts of the *tibias*, and *femurs*, and the *radii.*

167. A lesion that is hot on all 3 phases on a bone scan, can represent all, *except*:

a. osteomyelitis
b. tumor
c. neuropathic joint
d. chronic fracture
e. reflex sympathetic dystrophy

Answer: (D) Chronic fractures. All the other choices are correct.

168. (T/F) Radiotracer activity around a noncemented prosthesis can be seen for up to 6-12 months.

Answer: False. Radiotracer activity around a noncemented prosthesis can be seen for up to 24-36 months, and in a cemented prosthesis for 6-12 months. A loose hip prosthesis is suggested when there is increased activity near the lesser trochanter, and at the tip.

169. On a polar display of myocardial perfusion (bull's eye), the left portion of the map (ie. around the 3 o'clock region) correlates to which of the following?

a. left circumflex artery
b. right coronary artery
c. left anterior descending artery
d. septum
e. inferior wall

Answer: (A) The lateral wall is supplied by the left circumflex artery.

170. A rightward center of rotation error in cardiac SPECT imaging may result in a(n):

a. anteroapical defect
b. ring artifact
c. posteroapical defect
d. lateral defect
e. none of the above

Answer: (C) A rightward center of rotation error in cardiac SPECT imaging may result in a posteroapical defect.

171. (T/F) Reverse redistribution indicates stress-induced ischemia.

Answer: False. Reverse redistribution is seen when the delayed image shows a defect, but the poststress images are normal. Reverse redistribution has been associated with prior myocardial infarction. Its etiology is not definitively understood.

172. (T/F) On a cardiac thallium study, a large amount of splanchnic activity suggests submaximal exercise.

Answer: True. On a cardiac thallium study, a large amount of splanchnic activity suggests submaximal exercise. A paucity of activity suggests that significant exercise was achieved.

173. Which of the following is *not* a good cardiac protocol?

a. A rest 201-Thallium (3.5 mCi) dose, followed by stress 99m-Tc sestamibi study (20-30 mCi).
b. A dose of 99m-Tc sestamibi (5 mCi) at rest, and shortly followed by a 20 mCi dose of 99m-Tc sestamibi, for stress.
c. An injection of 20 mCi of 99m-Tc sestamibi for rest, followed the next day by an injection of 20 mCi of 99m-Tc sestamibi for stress.
d. Use of a low energy, all purpose collimator.
e. A rest 99m-Tc sestamibi study (20-30 mCi) injection, followed by a stress 201-Thallium (2.5 mCi) dose.

Answer: (E) The rest study is performed first with the *lower-energy* 201-Thallium, in order to prevent interference from 99m-Tc sestamibi, which is of higher energy.

174. Myocardial perfusion imaging in a patient with myocardial hypertrophy resulting from a long history of hypertension, may demonstrate relative increased activity in which wall?

a. Septum
b. Anterior wall
c. Lateral wall
d. Inferior wall
e. Antero-apex

Answer: (A) Myocardial perfusion imaging in a patient with myocardial hypertrophy resulting from a long history of hypertension, may demonstrate relative increased activity at the septum. This may show an apparent relative decrease in counts in the lateral wall.

175. Yttrium-90 ibritumomab tiuxetan (©Zevalin) is used for:

a. melanoma therapy
b. relapsed or refractory low-grade follicular non-Hodgkin's lymphoma
c. for preparation for Meckel's scan
d. patients who are CEA positive, but have a negative CT scan for colon carcinoma
e. Kaposi's sarcoma

Answer: (B) Yttrium-90 ibritumomab tiuxetan (Zevalin) offers an additional treatment option for patients with relapsed or refractory low-grade follicular non-Hodgkin's lymphoma. It is a radioimmunotherapy agent that combines imaging with therapy, utilizing a monoclonal antibody.

176. (T/F) MIBG is an analog for somatostatin.

Answer: False. Metaiodobenzylguanidine (MIBG) is an analog of guanethidine, which is taken up by an active amine transport mechanism. I-131 MIBG is used in neuroblastomas, paragangliomas, pheochromocytomas, and ganglioneuroblastomas. Indium-111-pentetreotide (© Octreoscan) is an analog of somatostatin. Octreoscan is used in neuroblastoma, medullary thyroid carcinoma, carcinoid, pheochromocytoma, and other neuroendocrine tumors.

177. (T/F) Heat damaged red blood cells are taken up by the spleen, but not by the marrow or the liver.

Answer: True. 99m-Tc damaged RBCs are useful for imaging splenic tissue, such as accessorry spleens, autotransplanted spleens in patients who have had splenectomy after trauma, and aberrant spleens.

178. (T/F) Bone scanning is a good method to evaluate bone graft viability.

Answer: True. A three phase bone scan is a good method in evaluating bone graft viability in a noninvasive manner. It will demonstrate increased radiotracer activity on all three phases. The activity will become more uniform to adjacent bone as the graft is incorporated.

179. (T/F) Eating solids before a renal captopril study is not recommended.

Answer: True. Patients should be NPO after midnight before the exam, since food may interfere with the absorption of captopril.

180. In PET, the unit measurements for the standard uptake value (SUV) is:

a. g/cm3
b. cm
c. g/liter
d. g/dl
e. it is unitless

Answer: (E) The standard uptake value is a unitless ratio, and is essentially the radiotracer concentration in the tumor, divided by the injected radiotracer concentration throughout the volume of the body.

181. Head and neck cancers constitute ___ of all newly diagnosed cancers. The majority of these cancers are ________.

a. 21%, adenocarcinoma
b. 12%, squamous carcinoma
c. 4%, squamous carcinoma
d. 2%, squamous carcinoma
e. 0.5%, adenocarcinoma

Answer: (C) 4%, squamous carcinoma.

182. 173. (T/F) PET scan results can be influenced by parenteral, but not oral antidiabetic therapy.

Answer: False. PET scan results can be influenced by *both* parenteral, and oral antidiabetic therapy. The sensitivity of PET decreases in hyperglycemic patients.

183. (T/F) In the detection of hepatic metastases from colorectal carcinoma, PET is roughly equal in sensitivity when compared with CT.

Answer: False. PET has superior sensitivity (approximately 90%) over CT (approximately 40%), in the detection of hepatic metastases.

184. (T/F) FDG-uptake is excellent for prostate cancer evaluation.

Answer: False. Prostate cancer, unlike most of the other common cancers, demonstrates a low proliferative activity. Therefore, it has unpredictable uptake. Prostate adenocarcinoma is often of the lower grade type.

185. In ovarian carcinoma, PET is less reliable than CEA assays for recurrence.

Answer: False. PET is more reliable than CEA assays for ovarian carcinoma recurrence.

186. The most common female genital cancer is:

a. endometrial
b. uterine
c. vaginal
d. cervical
e. ovarian

Answer: (A) The most common female genital cancer is endometrial carcinoma, which occurs in approximately 6-9% of all cancers in women. Risk factors include obesity, exogenous estrogen, and nulliparity.

187. With respect to the heart, Wenckebach phenomenon is:

a. The P-R gradually increases with each cycle, until the last P is not followed by a QRS
b. When the EKG strip demonstrates an occasional dropped QRS
c. A prolonged P-R interval greater than 0.2 seconds
d. When there is a block in a 2:1 AV pattern
e. When there is a block in a 3:1 AV pattern

Answer: (A) Wenckebach is when the P-R gradually increases with each cycle, until the last P is not followed by a QRS. Mobitz II is when some of the P's are not followed by a QRS, and may appear like an occasional dropped QRS.

188. If a source decays at 2% per hour, what is the $T_{1/2}$?

a. 12 hours
b. 20 hours
c. 24.8 hours
d. 35 hours
e. 69.3 hours

Answer: (D) $T_{1/2} = 0.693 / 2\% = 0.693 / 0.02 = 34.65$ hours.

189. There are 10 mCi of 99m-Tc at 10 am. What is the remaining activity at 7 pm?

a. 0.5 mCi
b. 3.5 mCi
c. 7.0 mCi
d. 7.5 mCi
e. 10.0 mCi

Answer: (B) $A_t = A_o\ (0.5)^{t\ /\ T\ 1/2} = 10\ (0.5)^{9/6} = 10 \times 0.35 = 3.5$ mCi.

190. (T/F) PET scanning is useful in renal cell carcinoma evaluation.

Answer: True. FDG is normally excreted by the kidneys, but PET scanning is still useful for renal cell carcinoma evaluation, provided the timing of the scan is appropriate.

191. 99m-Tc pertechnetate is physiologically seen in all, except:

a. choroid plexus
b. thyroid
c. small bowel
d. large bowel
e. liver

Answer: (E) 99m-Tc pertechnetate is physiologically seen in the stomach, bowel, salivary glands, choroid plexus, lactating breasts, kidneys, and thyroid gland. It is not physiologically seen in the liver.

192. (T/F) In PET imaging, bismuth germinate (BGO) crystals are less preferred than sodium iodide (NaI).

Answer: False. BGO crystals are preferred over NaI because they are more sensitive to 511 keV photons.

193. What are the number of counts required to produce a 2% uncertainty limit, and 95% confidence level?

a. 1,000
b. 2,000
c. 10,000
d. 20,000
e. 40,000

Answer: (C) $N = (n / uncertainty)^2$; n= #of standard deviations ; $N = (2 / 0.02)^2 = 10{,}000$.

194. In the cell cycle, which is the most resistant to radiation effects?

a. M
b. G2
c. G1
d. S

Answer: (D) The S phase is the most resistant.

195. The mechanism of localization of Tc-99m sulfur colloid is by:

a. active transport
b. capillary blockade
c. phagocytosis
d. compartmentalization
e. metabolic trapping

Answer: (C) The mechanism of localization of Tc-99m sulfur colloid is by phagocytosis. Thallium-201 acts by active transport. Tc-99m MAA is associated with capillary blockade. Tc-99m RBC is associated with compartmentalization, and FDG is by metabolic trapping.

196. 187. (T/F) In left bundle branch block, one can utilize adenosine or dypyridamole because they do not increase heart rate.

Answer: True. In left bundle branch block, one can utilize adenosine or dypyridamole because they do not increase heart rate.

197. (T/F) BEIR V indicates that the linear dose response model was best for all cancers, except for breast and prostate cancers.

Answer: False. BEIR V indicates that the linear dose response model was best for all cancers, except for bone cancer, and for leukemia. A linear-quadratic model was suggested for these two cancers.

198. (T/F) In computers, a word is often 8 bytes.

Answer: False. A Word is often associated with 2 or 4 bytes. A Bit is one binary digit. A Byte is 8 bits.

199. (T/F) With regard to the Poisson distribution, the variance is equal to the mean, and the standard deviation is equal to the square of the mean.

Answer: False. With regard to the Poisson distribution, the variance is equal to the mean, and the standard deviation is equal to the square *root* of the mean. The Poisson distribution is used to model radioactive decay.

200. (T/F) Free 99m-Tc migrates in saline, but not methanol.

Answer: False. Free 99m-Tc migrates in saline *and* methanol. 99m-Tc compounds migrate in saline only. These principles are utilized in radiochemical purity tests.

201. (T/F) 99m-Tc HMPAO is non-lipophilic.

Answer: False. 99m-Tc HMPAO is lipophilic and cross the blood-brain barrier. The other brain agents, glucoheptanate, pertechnetate, and DTPA are non-lipophilic and will cross the blood-brain barrier, if damaged.

202. Patients at higher risk for thyroid storm after I-131 therapy include all, except:

a. patients with severe thyrotoxicosis
b. patients placed on a beta blocker
c. the elderly
d. those with underlying heart disease

Answer: (B) Thyroid storm, a rare occurrence, may occur 1-2 weeks following I-131 therapy, due to release of stored hormones. Thyroid storm is a severe life-threatening form of hyperthyroidism.

203. (T/F) The 24-hour uptake will be high in a patient with hyperthyroidism secondary to struma ovarii.

Answer: False. This very rare conditions is due to an ovarian teratoma or adenomatous thyroid tissue, which suppresses the normal thyroid gland. The 24-hour uptake will be low, close to zero. The pelvis should be imaged if this condition is suspected.

204. (T/F) Approximately 5% of hyperthyroid patients need to be retreated with I-131 therapy.

Answer: False. About 10-20% of Graves' disease patients may need a second dose.

205. (T/F) Bone scans are highly sensitive and specific for arthritis.

Answer: False. Bone scan are sensitive, but *not* specific for arthritis. Arthritis often yields diffuse periarticular uptake.

206. (T/F) The patient should be without food (NPO) for at least 4 hours before a bone scan.

Answer: False. There is no special preparation for a bone scan. However, the patient should drink liberally before and after the procedure. The patient should also void often, since most of the radiotracer is excreted through the urine.

207. Falsely elevated measurements in bone DXA (densitometry) studies can be due to the following, except:

a. degenerative changes
b. vascular calcifications
c. tumors
d. inclusion of ribs in the region of interest
e. laminectomy

Answer: (E) Laminectomy will often yield lower bone mineral density values.

208. A 64 year old female with a left femoral neck composite bone mineral density of 0.799, a T-score of -1.39, and a z-score of -0.31 is (assuming that the T-score in the lumbar spine is -1.40, and the z-score is -0.41):

a. normal
b. osteopenic
c. osteoporotic
d. none of the above

Answer: (B) Osteopenic. According to the WHO, a T-score between -1 to -2.5 is defined as osteopenic, while below (or equal to) -2.5, it is osteoporotic.

209. A single photopenic defect in a colloid liver scan can be seen in the following, except:

a. cyst
b. hemangioma
c. single metastasis
d. amyloid
e. subphrenic abscess

Answer: (D) Amyloid is associated with *diffuse* photopenic areas.

Interesting and Useful Websites

1. American Board of Nuclear Medicine
   www.abnm.org

2. American College of Radiology
   www.acr.org

3. American Society of Nuclear Cardiology
   www.asnc.org

4. American Board of Radiology
   www.theabr.org

5. Society of Nuclear Medicine
   www.snm.org

6. Mallinkrodt Institute of Radiology Teaching Files
   http://gamma.wustl.edu/home.html

7. The Journal of Nuclear Medicine
   http://jnm.snmjournals.org

8. Harvard Medical School Joint Program in Nuclear Medicine
   www.jpnm.org

9. Auntminnie.com
   www.auntminnie.com

10. National Council on Radiation Protection and Measurements
    www.ncrp.com

11. Radiological Society of North America (RSNA)
    www.rsna.org

References

1. Habibian MR, Delbeke D, Martin WH, Sandler MO: Nuclear Medicine Imaging – A Teaching File, Philadelphia, 1999, Lippincott Williams & Wilkins.

2. Maisy MM, Wahl RL, Barrington SF: Atlas of Clinical Positron Emission Tomography, New York, 1999, Oxford University Press Inc.

3. Mettler FA, Guiberteau MJ: Essentials of Nuclear Medicine Imaging, ed 4, Philadelphia, 1998, W.B. Saunders Company.

4. Saha GB: Fundamentals of Nuclear Pharmacy, ed 4, New York, 1998, Springer-Verlag.

5. Thrall JH, Ziessman HA: Nuclear Medicine – The Requisites, ed 2, St Louis, 2001, Mosby.

6. Weissleder R, Rieumont MJ, Wittenberg J: Primer of Diagnostic Imaging, ed 2, St Louis, 1997, Mosby.

7. Ziessman HA, Rehm P: Nuclear Medicine – Case Review, St Louis, 2002, Mosby.

The books listed in the references are invaluable, excellent sources, and are recommended for further reading.

Made in the USA
Monee, IL
08 November 2026

67378655R00037